# The Truth
# About Getting Sick
# in America

# The Truth About Getting Sick in America

The Real Problems with Health Care
and What We Can Do

## Dr. Tim Johnson

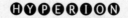

NEW YORK

ISBN: 978-1-4013-1087-5

Hyperion books are available for special
promotions and premiums. For details
contact the HarperCollins Special Markets
Department in the New York office at
212-207-7528, fax 212-207-7222, or email
spsales@harpercollins.com.

First Paperback Edition
10 9 8 7 6 5 4 3 2

# Acknowledgments

It has become a cliché, but in this case it is absolutely true: This book would not have been possible without the spectacular help of several friends and colleagues.

First and foremost, I thank Dr. Mark Abdelmalek, currently a dermatologist and faculty member at the Drexel University College of Medicine in Philadelphia. I first met Mark when he interned in our ABC News office in Boston. He immediately distinguished himself as a brilliant researcher and thinker about anything medical, including health care policy. He has held my hand throughout the writing of this book and written the section on Germany. Put simply, I could not have done this without Mark.

I also wish to thank my ABC News colleague Jay Shaylor for writing about the Federal Employees Health Benefits (FEHB) program. Jay was my producer when I did a fascinating report about the Office of the Attending Physician to Congress and was fearless in researching this hidden jewel in the basement of the U.S. Capitol.

Stephanie Young has been my wonderful editor and Elizabeth Sabo our guide at Hyperion. I could not have found two more delightful people to work with.

And, finally, I thank my wife Nancy for putting up with me, once again, as I have given birth to another book, this one in less than nine months.

# Contents

# Introduction

"We Americans have the best health care in the world." That's what many politicians tell us. And if you are (a) wealthy, (b) well insured, and/or (c) have the right connections, you have probably experienced the truth of that statement. But many of us also know people who do not fall into those categories and who have had great difficulty in getting timely, quality medical care.

And as a result of the ongoing and heated debate about health care reform, we also hear that other countries have health care just as good as ours, provide health insurance to all their citizens—*and* do so at a significantly lower cost. So what is the truth? Do we Americans really have "the best health care in the world"? And if we truly have the best, why does it need reform?

Alas, when the subject of reform comes up, we usually find ourselves awash in a tsunami of political posturing and caustic catchphrases, such as "government takeover," "market mayhem," or "death panels"—all of which are calculated to scare the daylights out of us, so we stop thinking about the underlying issues. But we need to start thinking and start talking. I recognize that for most Americans, finding out "the truth" about current problems or possible fixes is virtually impossible amid all the emotionally charged rhetoric. If you're in that camp, I would like to reach out and help you.

I have reported on health for ABC News part-time since 1975, when I joined a new program called *Good Morning America*, and full-time since 1984, when I became the Medical Editor of ABC News. Until the late 1990s, the majority of my time was spent on reporting and commenting about new developments in clinical medicine (such as an innovative technique for treating heart disease or a new drug for cancer) and promoting old ideas for good health (such as the importance of good nutrition and regular exercise).

But as we all entered this new century, I became increasingly concerned about the major problems with the way we Americans often receive and pay for our health care. Clearly, some of us *have* been blessed to receive the best care available anywhere in the world. However, because we don't have anything that could be called a national "system" of health care in this country, many Americans are falling between the cracks and not getting any care—or getting care that is either inferior or too costly or both.

We do have many mini-systems of health care and insurance programs in this country, such as private medical systems like the Cleveland or Mayo clinics, or public insurance programs like Medicare or Medicaid. However, there is no *national* system that binds them together in a working whole. And when you're scrambling to find health care insurance you can afford—when you or a spouse lose a job or when your company decides it can no longer afford health insurance— you are faced with the reality that there is no *national* plan as a backup or replacement.

During this past decade at ABC News, I began to realize that it was just as important for me to report and talk about health care system problems as about new medical developments. Lack of health insurance can be just as deadly as lack of antibiotics, because people with no insurance often delay in getting needed medical care.

I also began to realize that most Americans (myself included) had no idea how costly and complicated our health care had become, and how often politicians used rhetoric that was either deliberately misleading or downright false. So I decided that I had to start talking and writing about health care in the same way I have reported on medical discoveries all these years: with honesty and using terms that people could understand. *And*, quite frankly, I am also motivated to do this on behalf of my children and grandchildren, because they are going to face disaster if we don't fix the current problems with American health care.

That's why I have spent increasing amounts of my professional time studying health care in America. And I would like to share with you the most important insights I have gained. Here is an overview.

**Chapter One: The Big Question:** First, I will explore the exploding costs of American health care and whether or not we get full value for the money we spend. In this chapter, and throughout the book, I will try to pinpoint the factors that have driven up U.S. health care costs higher and faster than in other developed countries.

**Chapter Two: The Big Problem:** What's the biggest obstacle to health care reform in this country? One of them is certainly our unrealistic expectations as to what our health care can and should do. To put it bluntly, most of us want a gourmet platter of care and services at a blue-plate-special price. And, all too often, we expect top-notch results without any personal effort to improve what we can about our health through such proven techniques as regular exercise or improved nutrition.

I'll illustrate how those expectations translate into the current gridlock in Congress, and why our politicians don't dare limit care and/or increase costs for the voters who elect them. This chapter will also introduce the big players—hospitals, doctors, insurers, lawyers, drug and medical device companies, and the media—who create and contribute to the reform traffic jam. Also, I'll begin to explore the devastating effects of the growing lack of primary care in our country.

**Chapter Three: The Big Fear:** According to many experts, any truly effective control of costs and improvement in quality in American health care would require more government regulation. But in the current political environment, which plays off understandable fears about "big government" in general and "government takeover" of health care in particular, that idea seems less and less palatable. Nevertheless, I will describe an industry in this country that might serve as a model for a sensible partnership between government and private industry. I will also discuss how the federal government of another major developed country plays an essential role in health care, and how we might learn from that country.

**Chapter Four: The Big Sermon:** Is health care a right or a privilege? Is there any moral obligation for our nation to provide health care to all? In this chapter I will put on my ministerial collar—I am also an ordained Protestant minister—and explore some of the teachings from my own religious tradition that might speak to these questions.

**Chapter Five: The Big Prediction:** Here, I will be brutally honest in predicting what I think will actually happen to our health care in the long term and what would be needed to truly control costs and improve quality.

Throughout the book, I will also discuss how some of the ideas in the new Patient Protection and Affordable Care Act (usually described by opponents as ObamaCare) might affect our future health care. I will not go into an in-depth analysis of that new legislation, because most of the details will certainly change over time. In other words, this book is about essential principles rather than policy details.

My intent is to be as honest as humanly possible about the problems we face with American health care. I have no political axe to grind. I am independent in my political judgments; I vote for the person, not the party. Yes, like any human being, I do have opinions, even biases. But I hope they are informed by facts and figures, not by fables or fiction. You will have to decide for yourself. Now that I am no longer the full-time Medical Editor of ABC News, I can more freely express my opinions on this vital subject.

My goal is to help you understand what I think are some of the most important issues that need to be addressed by any honest proposals to reform our health care. I hope to foster a dialogue that will get all of us—whatever our particular political or social opinions—talking seriously about how we can help to solve the problems we face. So let's get going.

# The Truth
# About Getting Sick
# in America

# CHAPTER ONE

# The Big Question

I begin with what I believe is the most important question that needs to be asked (and answered) if we are ever going to make the right changes for health care in our country. So here it is:

WHY DOES THE UNITED STATES SPEND MORE THAN *TWICE AS MUCH* PER PERSON ON HEALTH CARE AS THE AVERAGE PER PERSON COST FOR ALL OTHER INDUSTRIALIZED COUNTRIES EVEN THOUGH IT IS STILL *THE ONLY DEVELOPED COUNTRY* THAT DOESN'T PROVIDE BASIC HEALTH INSURANCE FOR ALL ITS CITIZENS?

Think about it: twice as much per person as the average of all industrialized nations. How does that translate into dollars? Let's look at the health care spending in some other industrialized nations. According to a 2010 Organization for Economic Co-operation and Development Report, and 2009 National Health expenditure data from the Centers for Medicare & Medicaid Services, the five highest and the five lowest per person spenders were:

### Top 5 Spenders

| | |
|---|---|
| United States* | $8086 |
| Norway** | $5003 |
| Switzerland* | $4810 |
| Canada* | $4406 |
| Luxembourg** | $4237 |

## Bottom 5 Spenders

| | |
|---|---|
| Turkey** | $818 |
| Mexico* | $877 |
| Chile** | $999 |
| Poland** | $1213 |
| Hungary** | $1437 |

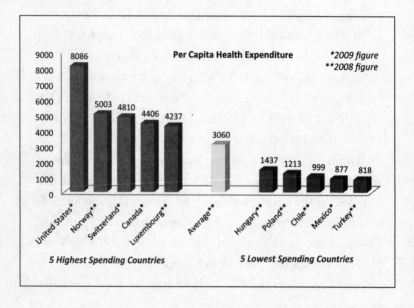

As you can see, there is quite a range from the United States at the top to Turkey at the bottom, but the 2008 per capita average among all industrialized countries was $3,060—and we spend more than twice that! And since these numbers were gathered, our spending has only continued to rise. In 2011, CMS projects the overall cost of health care in the United States at $8643 per person.

This high per-person cost means a frightening upward spiral: The *total* cost for health care in this country in 2011 will be about $2.7 trillion—more than 17 percent of our GDP. Recent numbers from the Milliman Medical Index show that health care for the average American family now costs more than $18,000 a year in insurance premiums (from both employer and employee) plus deductibles paid by the family. During the decade from 1999 to 2009, the inflation rate for health care grew 60 percent faster than the general inflation rate! And during this same decade, health insurance premiums rose an average of 13 percent per year!

If these trends continue, the average cost of health insurance for a family of four will double in the next ten years to more than $25,000 per year and health care will consume about 20 percent of our GDP, at a cost of more than $13,000 per person! That would leave very little discretionary money for other vital national needs like education and infrastructure (bridges, roads, etc.). No wonder experts say we are headed for individual and national bankruptcy if we don't get costs under control! As Warren Buffett chillingly put it, health care costs are like "a tapeworm eating at our economic body."

What do we get for all that spending? Better health care? Health care that's twice as good? Obviously, "good" is a vague term, but most experts would start to answer such questions by looking at outcomes, or results. So let's look at three ways to measure outcomes.

One straightforward way is life expectancy: Either someone is dead or not. Again using the latest report from the Organization for Economic Co-operation and Development, comparing life expectancy rates for the higher health-spending countries, we find:

## Life Expectancy in the Top 5 Spenders

| | |
|---|---|
| United States*** | 77.9 years |
| Norway** | 80.6 years |
| Switzerland** | 82.2 years |
| Canada** | 80.7 years |
| Luxembourg** | 80.6 years |

## Life Expectancy in the Bottom 5 Spenders

| | |
|---|---|
| Turkey** | 73.6 years |
| Mexico* | 75.3 years |
| Chile* | 78.1 years |
| Poland** | 75.6 years |
| Hungary** | 73.8 years |

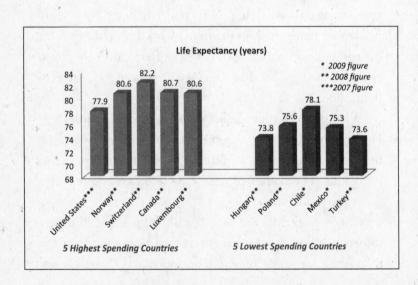

A quick scan of the numbers shows that the United States does *not* do twice as well; it actually has the *lowest* life expectancy of the top spenders!

So Americans don't live as long, but is the American health care system to blame? Some argue life expectancy is not a fair reflection on the quality of a nation's health care. After all, tens of thousands of people die in car accidents or are murdered every year, and that has nothing to do with health care. So yet another way to look at mortality numbers is to look at "amenable mortality."

This figure represents the number of deaths (age seventy-five or less per one hundred thousand population) that are potentially preventable by a nation's health care system. Some experts say it's a better indicator of the quality of a nation's health care system than raw mortality numbers. The Commonwealth Fund, a private organization that studies health policy, funded a study published in *Health Affairs* in 2008 to compare our amenable mortality rate to that of eighteen other industrialized nations. How did we do? We came in first, but not in a good way.

**Best (Lowest) Rates**

| | |
|---|---|
| France | 65 |
| Japan and Australia | 71 |
| Spain and Italy | 74 |
| Canada | 77 |
| Norway | 80 |

### Worst (Highest) Rates

| | |
|---|---|
| United States | 110 |
| Portugal | 104 |
| United Kingdom and Ireland | 103 |
| Denmark | 101 |
| New Zealand | 96 |

As if having the worst amenable mortality rate weren't enough, the Commonwealth Study concluded that 101,000 deaths could have been prevented in 2002–2003 had America's health care system performed as well as the average rate of the three top performing countries.

Disease data is a third way to compare mortality numbers; in other words, looking at survival rates for diseases common to industrialized countries, such as cancers or heart disease. In this case, instead of the world, let's narrow the comparison to our northern neighbor, since the current health care debate so often points to the contrasts between the United States and Canada. The following numbers come from the 2009 reports published independently by the American and Canadian cancer societies. These reports show Americans having slightly higher five-year survival rates for eight of the reported cancer types, Canadians having slightly higher survival rates for seven cancer types, and Americans and Canadians having essentially the same rates for two cancer types.

### Where the U.S. Does Better

Breast (88.7%-U.S. vs. 87%-CA)
Colorectal (64.4%-U.S. vs. 62%-CA)

Esophageal (15.8%-U.S. vs. 14%-CA)

Melanoma (91.2%-U.S. vs. 89%-CA)

Ovarian (45.5%-U.S. vs. 40%-CA)

Prostate (98.9%-U.S. vs. 95%-CA)

Stomach (24.7%-U.S. vs. 23%-CA)

Bladder (79.8%-U.S. vs. 77%-CA)

### Where Canada Does Better

Laryngeal (65%-CA vs. 62.5%-U.S.)

Liver (18%-CA vs. 11.7%-U.S.)

Oral cavity and pharyngeal (63%-CA vs. 59.7%-U.S.)

Pancreatic (6%-CA vs. 5.1%-U.S.)

Testicular (96%-CA vs. 95.5%-U.S.)

Thyroid (98%-CA vs. 96.9%-U.S.)

Cervical (75%-CA vs. 71.2%-U.S.)

### Where There's a Tie

Kidney (66.5%-U.S. vs. 66%-CA)

Lung (15.2%-U.S. vs. 15%- CA)

The take-home message: While the two countries are very similar in cancer treatment outcomes, there are certainly no "twice as good" numbers, even though we spend almost twice as much per person on health care as Canada ($8086 in the United States compared to $4406 in Canada annually.)

While we're on the subject of America and Canada, I want to tell you a story about the first time my own eyes were really opened to the possibility that other developed countries might have something to teach us about how to improve our own health care delivery. Back in the early

1990s, I was asked by the late Peter Jennings, then anchor of *World News Tonight*, to do a four-minute report comparing the U.S. and Canadian health care systems. It sounded impossible to accomplish in such a short time, but we eventually came up with an idea that was quite dramatic and revealing.

We called the family practice organization in the state of New York and asked them to pick a typical two-physician practice in their state; we then asked the similar organization in the province of Ontario, just over the border, to do the same. Then we asked each practice to pick a young family with two parents and two young children that we could interview.

First we went to the practice in New York. During the course of our interviews, I was shocked to learn that the practice employed several full-time persons to do nothing but the insurance billing because there were so many different companies and forms to deal with!

When we interviewed the young family, we learned that the husband was a self-employed logger who made slightly too much to qualify for Medicaid but not enough to afford health insurance. So when their six-month-old child had been born, the father had to sit in the business office to negotiate a long-term payment plan while his wife was in labor!

Across the border in Canada, we learned that the two-physician practice had someone come in just ten hours a week to fill out insurance forms, because it was the same form for everyone. The government was the single payer for all claims, even though the doctors and hospitals were private. And when I interviewed the young Canadian family, the husband described what happened during the birth of their youngest child: He said, "I showed them our card [the government insurance card] and they whisked us upstairs."

Actually, the Canadian system is virtually the same as Medicare in *this* country: The government is the single insurer but patients can choose the doctors/hospitals they want. It is true that Canadians often have longer waits for non-emergency services and some choose to go outside the country to avoid those waits. But as the cancer statistics we have just seen show, there really is no difference between the United States and Canada on mortality outcomes.

So if we can't explain our higher per-person costs with various mortality data, what about some other justifications for our higher health care price tag? One common claim is that even if mortality statistics don't clearly show it, by spending more on doctors and hospitals, we get better quality of life, if not better mortality outcomes. It's natural to assume that if you spend more, you'll get a better product. That basic concept may be largely true in the food, clothing, and housing industries, but it looks like it's not always true in medical care.

Researchers at Dartmouth College have been looking into this matter for almost two decades and they conclude that in medicine, "more isn't always better."

Most of the Dartmouth studies are based on Medicare spending. For example, the researchers found that costs for a Medicare patient in Miami is a lot more expensive than in

Iowa City, Iowa, or Salem, Oregon. Take a look at the dramatic differences:

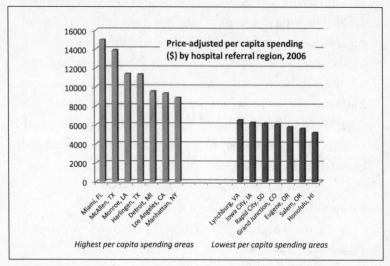

Source: D. Gottlieb et al., "Prices Don't Drive Regional Medicare Spending Variations," *Health Affairs* 29 (March 2010): 3.

Since the basic Medicare payment rates (price-adjusted to compensate for cost-of-living differences) are the same, higher per-person costs mean that each person is actually getting more care, in the form of more tests, more surgeries, etc. But is the person better off for it?

In 2003, in an *Annals of Internal Medicine* study, Dartmouth researchers compared Medicare spending across the country for heart attack, hip fracture, and colorectal cancer patients, and found that in the highest-spending areas (mid-Atlantic region), patients received 60 percent more care than patients in the lowest-spending areas (Great Plains or Pacific). Patients in the higher-spending areas went to the doctor more

often, saw more specialists, had more tests and minor procedures, and were hospitalized more often than those in lower-
spending areas. So did those who received 60 percent more
care do better than those who received less care? Surprisingly,
the answer was *no*.

Overall, higher spending did *not* result in improved survival, a slower decline in functional status, or improved patient satisfaction. In fact, the researchers found that patients
in the highest-spending regions had a slightly higher relative
risk of death than those in the lower-spending ones.

Now that we understand that American health care costs
so much more but is basically no better in outcomes, it is
time to look at factors that we can relate to in a more personal way than statistical comparisons between industrialized nations. As Shakespeare once famously suggested, it may
be that the fault is within ourselves!

# CHAPTER TWO

# The Big Problem

A significant driver of cost in any social service, such as health care, is the demand for that service. When it comes to health care, we Americans seem to have an insatiable appetite for high-level care. I call these collective demands the four "C's." We want health care that is:

1. **Convenient:** We are usually impatient when it comes to something we want or think we need. We have been trained to be impulse buyers, so we can't wait. Health care is no exception. If we think we are sick, we want an appointment with the best doctor as soon as possible, preferably at a nearby facility with free parking, thank you!

2. **Compassionate, Communicative, Coordinated:** Who wouldn't want this kind of health care? Especially when we are sick, we want to be treated with tender loving care topped by a tincture of boundless time. We want care where "everyone knows our name" and they all work together on our behalf.

3. **Cutting Edge:** We have become convinced that the newest drugs, devices, tests, and scans are automatically the best. So we tend to demand what we have read about on the Internet and heard about (the media love to talk about cutting edge discoveries and medical miracles—good for ratings).

**4. Cheap—or even better, Cost-free:** We have been brought up with the expectation that somebody else should and will provide health care. For the majority of us, it has been our employer. For many of us, it has increasingly been some form of government (state and/or federal) insurance. But whether or not we truly believe that health care is a right (see Chapter 4) most of us believe that the cost of health care should somehow be mostly borne by our society and, if necessary, its government. (I have always thought that this is partly due to a subconscious objection to paying for something we didn't want or ask for—getting sick. In our heads, we know that good health care has to be paid for, but in our hearts, we don't think it should be us as individuals doing the paying.)

Now, there is nothing inherently wrong with these expectations. But to demand this kind of care without worrying about how to pay for it? That's *not* sensible or responsible. Whatever the historical and sociological origins of the American palate for gourmet health care services, that expectation has become a persistent and pernicious push for more goods and services willingly offered by a vast array of providers, sometimes characterized as the "medical-industrial complex."

That phrase derives from the infamous "military-industrial complex" described in 1961, by then-President Dwight Eisenhower, as a looming force that would lead to out-of-control expenditures in defense spending. And while the end products and services are very different in health care than in defense, the underlying economic dynamics are often similar.

Both defense and health industries operate very much in

the shadows of hidden costs (and, by the way, we spend more than three times as much on health care as on defense). It is extremely difficult for us as consumers of health care to know what the real costs are because the billings of providers are virtually incomprehensible. And that makes it easy to slip in such things as $640 toilet seats in the defense budget or $10 aspirin tablets in a hospital bill. But these two industries are similar in another way—their incentivized spending—that is even more threatening to the economic bottom line in health care.

Our present health care reimbursement systems are based primarily on paying for procedures rather than for results or outcomes. It is much easier to bill for specific tests, surgeries, scans, biopsies, drugs, etc., than to charge according to outcomes, e.g., how a patient does, which can be nebulous and take a long time to determine. That's why, when you see a bill from a doctor or hospital, it lists all kinds of procedures and products. It is much harder to figure out how to charge for "thinking time"—all the important moments health professionals should be using to contemplate, discuss, and decide what is really best for the patient rather than simply ordering more tests and procedures. To put it bluntly, our current payment system boils down to a simple yet ultimately disastrous financial incentive: *The more you do, the more you make.*

And if we consumers have no financial skin in the game, we have no reason not to ask for the latest and newest medical miracles. This perverse combination of *provider incentive* (which can easily spill over into pure greed) and *consumer desire* often plays out most dramatically for Medicare patients. Because of their age and worries about declining health, they are often at the mercy of a given provider, who in turn simply drives up costs by doing more. Such doctors and hospitals are understandably attracted to areas where large numbers of Medicare patients live. That's one reason our government spends almost three times as much per Medicare patient in Miami, Florida, as it does in Salem, Oregon—with no difference in outcomes.

One of the reasons patient costs can easily soar out of control is that there is often no single doctor in charge. In "the good old days," most people had a family doctor, typically a general practitioner (GP), who took care of the whole family, knew them personally and was easily able to determine what might be best for them. Today, health care is saturated with specialists who often don't communicate with one another, order tests that have already been done, and prescribe medicines without knowing what else the patient is taking. That's one reason 20 percent of Medicare patients consume 70 percent of Medicare dollars; complicated patients amplify the inefficiencies and wastefulness that result when there's no one in charge. (In Chapter 5, I will discuss what we need to do about this growing imbalance between generalists—today called primary care doctors—and specialists.)

But the dearth of primary care isn't the only reason for growing costs. The following chart, from the Centers for Medicare and Medicaid Services, shows where our health care dollars go.

And since the majority of these dollars go to physicians and hospitals, I am going to start with them and then move on to four other critical drivers of health care costs in this country.

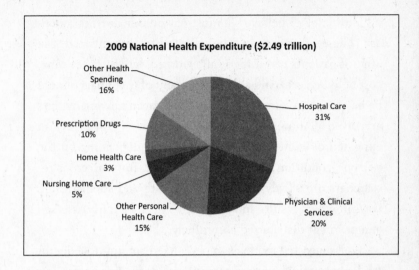

**2009 National Health Expenditure ($2.49 trillion)**

Other Health Spending 16%

Prescription Drugs 10%

Home Health Care 3%

Nursing Home Care 5%

Other Personal Health Care 15%

Hospital Care 31%

Physician & Clinical Services 20%

## DOCTORS

Between charges for their own professional services and the costs they produce by ordering tests, prescriptions, scans, surgeries, etc., doctors control as much as two-thirds of our health care dollars. This is one factor that makes health care unique among most other segments of the economy: Doctors are able to create demand for their services simply because of their near-absolute autonomy over diagnosis and treatment. So the forces that determine how much and what kind of medical services are ordered by doctors are still the single most important factor in driving up health care costs.

That's why I have come to believe that the most critical factor in true reform will depend on the success we have in changing the way we pay our doctors and hospitals.

Ultimately, I believe we must pay all our doctors by salary. These salaries should be adjusted for patient load, the kind of patients cared for, hours worked, length of training, cost of living, etc. And a key component of that salary should be based on outcomes. By that, I don't mean how many lives are saved or how healthy patients become. Obviously, an expected outcome will vary enormously depending on the person's condition and age to begin with. But outcomes researchers are slowly developing accurate and sophisticated ways in which results and productivity can be fairly assessed and payment distributed accordingly.

One suggested model is to pay a fixed amount to a doctor (and a hospital when such care is needed) for a given patient, based on that patient's age, existing medical conditions, family history, etc. If that patient—or a whole group of patients under the care of a given doctor—does better than expected and costs less money, the doctor might actually keep the difference, a kind of bonus. Similarly, if the patient does worse than expected and costs more money, the doctor may lose money. Now obviously this must be based on long-term results where the incentive is not to spend as little as possible but instead is to spend as much as necessary for good results—but not for extra care that is not really necessary and (in the case of dangerous tests or surgeries, for example) might actually produce worse outcomes. In addition to a base salary, there can also be financial incentives for doing screenings or immunizations that are proven to be cost-effective.

Currently, some of our best health care facilities, such

as the Mayo and Cleveland clinics, pay their doctors by salary in order to free them up from making decisions based on how much more money they could make. And if you combine this kind of payment reform with other reforms such as computer systems that eliminate most paperwork, paying off student loans, and minimizing medical malpractice threats, I predict that the vast majority of young physicians would choose to work on salary—*if* the salary is fair and adequate.

Fairness must include modifying the currently distorted disparities between specialists who can charge more for complicated procedures (such as heart and orthopedic surgeons) and primary care specialists (such as general internists, pediatricians, and family physicians) who don't do such procedures but constantly make decisions that will have a profound impact on the long-term health and cost for a given patient.

I am not saying that all doctors should be paid the same without regard to specialty. I believe that doctors who perform complicated, tension-filled procedures requiring longer training should be paid more than physicians who work under less stressful situations and/or have shorter training. But the differences should be less than they are today. In the following box ("How Much Should Doctors Make?"), I propose salary ranges for these two groups.

## HOW MUCH SHOULD DOCTORS MAKE?

**1. Primary Care Doctors:** $200,000–$300,000/year. This group includes family physicians (trained to take care of the entire family), pediatricians (for kids), and general internists (for adults.) All three require a three-year training program (residency) after medical school—for a total of seven years after college. This range would accommodate factors such as local cost of living, stage of career, type of patients, hours worked, etc. And because these kinds of physicians are so necessary to good health care, I think they should be able to reach the upper end of this salary range sooner rather than later.

**2. Procedural Physicians:** $300,000–$500,000/year. This group includes everyone from surgeons (who, by definition, do procedures) to non-surgeons whose practices are often filled with procedures (radiologists, cardiologists, gastroenterologists, etc.). The training time for these specialists is longer than for primary care doctors—usually two to five years longer, for a total of nine to twelve years after college. I have suggested this wide range to account for the diversity of practice conditions. So, for example, a neurosurgeon who does long, complicated brain procedures most days of the week would be on the high end of this range, while a neurosurgeon who no longer does surgery but sees patients in this office full-time might have very similar working conditions and hours to a family physician and therefore should be paid similarly.

Feeling some sticker shock over my numbers? For those of you who think they are too high, I remind you of the very long years (and hours) of training required after college for doctors. Put bluntly, $500,000 for a neurosurgeon with twelve years' training after college looks paltry compared to the multimillion-dollar bonuses for Wall Street traders with only four years of college. And for those of you who think my salary suggestions are too low, I would say that making big money should never be the primary motivation for the physicians we want taking care of us and our families.

Salaries have the advantage of eliminating the inherent conflict of interest in our fee-for-service system, which provides a direct financial incentive to do more. That incentive becomes even more intense with other kinds of conflict of interest, such as physicians owning medical facilities with scanning machines, for example, to which they can refer their own patients. I believe such conflicts of interest must be carefully controlled with full disclosure. In fact, I would prefer to see them totally eliminated.

However, we must also provide a pathway for physician-scientists and research-entrepreneurs that leads to important new discoveries. How this can be done without financial conflict of interest that leads to tainted choices for patient care is an issue hospitals and medical schools wrestle with daily. The general principle must be to isolate such activity from these conflicts of interest where patients are involved. However, physicians wishing to pursue an entrepreneurial path should be allowed to reap the rewards of taking their own financial risks.

## HOSPITALS

Many of the same financial dynamics described above for doctors apply to most hospitals: The more they do, the more they make! In fact, this distorted incentive often binds doctors and hospitals into the same money-making dynamics: Hospitals want to attract the doctors who can do the procedures that make big money for both! That's why there is often fierce competition for cardiologists who do angioplasties and orthopedic surgeons who do hip replacements and radiologists who do surgical-like procedures.

There is also competition among hospitals, especially in large cities with many major medical centers, for the latest technologies that can both bring in big bucks and attract (or keep) the doctors who perform these procedures. Stop and think of all the ads you hear on the radio (and see on billboards, TV, and in newspapers and magazines) trumpeting the latest machine that "Mount Olympus" or "Saint Miraculous" hospital has just acquired—and without which you are clearly destined to die. In fact, this medical arms race *would* be humorous if it weren't for the spiraling costs and the resulting danger to patients who are seduced into having risky procedures they really don't need.

I should say a special word about so-called "teaching hospitals"—the hospitals that also provide training to medical students and residents as they become our future doctors. As we try to control costs for all hospitals, including teaching hospitals, we need to be careful to preserve funding for this vital training function.

Once again, the ultimate answer is to figure out how to

pay hospitals for what works and what is really necessary. And because big hospitals today are usually part of some kind of system that also includes doctors, outpatient clinics, etc.—sometimes with their own insurance program to market these products—any cost control will have to involve all parts of the system. That is a topic I will cover in the next chapter.

## DRUG AND DEVICE COMPANIES

Pharmaceutical and device manufacturers are driven by the same intense competition to attract consumers to high-profit products. (For practical purposes, I am going to focus on drugs, but devices are quite similar in their marketplace dynamics.) Watch television or read just about any newspaper or magazine and you'll see advertisements for the *newest* (and therefore presumably the *best*) medication to hit the market. These glossy ads obviously add to the cost of the product.

But is the new medication better than the ones we already have now? Well, the drug companies certainly want you to think so, and they work hard to convince you *and* your doctor that this is the truth. (Remember, all these ads end with the seemingly benign phrase "Ask your doctor if 'Miracle X' is right for you.") This is also why, when you are at your doctor's office complaining about a nagging back pain or headache, your doctor may hand you a bunch of free samples that the pharmaceutical rep has dropped off. It's another, and often very effective, way of getting you to use a particular drug.

But new is not necessarily improved, meaning more effective or more safe. Time reveals the truth better than any advertisement or promotion can. In a 2002 issue of the *Journal of the American Medical Association*, researchers predicted that the probability of a new drug being pulled off the market for safety reasons or receiving a black box warning (the strongest warning the FDA can give) over a twenty-five-year period was 20 percent!

You probably remember the blockbuster drug Vioxx, touted as superior to existing anti-inflammatory pain medications such as Motrin or Advil. It was initially approved for a rather small group of people whose stomachs could not tolerate the traditional medications. Soon, it was being heavily promoted in extensive public advertising that quickly paid off. In the five years Vioxx was on the market, 100 million prescriptions were written in the United States alone, and Vioxx sales were estimated at $2.5 billion every year Vioxx was on the market!

But in 2004, this new drug was pulled off the market (after being linked, in this particular case, to fatal heart attacks and strokes). The FDA's initial estimate was that Vioxx caused almost 28,000 heart attacks and sudden cardiac deaths in the first four years it was on the market.

In order to control drug and device costs, we must have better ways of studying them for effectiveness and safety before they get approved and unleashed in the marketplace.

I also favor a ban on public advertising until a new drug has been in the marketplace for at least two years; that would provide more time to reveal safety and/or effectiveness issues that didn't show up during the limited testing done for FDA approval. That also means we have to beef up the post-approval surveillance resources at the FDA to keep track of problems with new drugs after approval.

## INSURERS

I certainly am no defender of the insurance companies, especially the for-profit ones that must return a profit to stockholders and often pay huge salaries and bonuses to their executives. These companies are basically middlemen, using dollars from our premiums to pay for their overhead—dollars which therefore don't go to actual health care. To be fair, their average profit margins (about 3–4 percent) are relatively small compared to other industries. But the moral question is whether there should be *any* profit when it comes to something as vital as delivering health care. And when these companies use truly appalling techniques—rescinding care because of a technicality or denying coverage due to preexisting conditions while trying to enroll young healthy customers less likely to dig into their profits—they resemble vultures, preying on the sick and vulnerable. (These kinds of insurance practices are one of the targets of the new health care bill, and these are changes which most Americans, of all political stripes, approve.)

But having said all this, I also have some sympathy for insurance companies, which are often caught between the proverbial rock and a hard place. On the one hand, they must try to meet the unrealistic expectations of all of us consumers who want the newest, the latest, the most expensive care at no or little cost. On the other, they must fight off the constantly increasing demands of their providers (doctors and hospitals) for higher payments. In very simple terms: We want our insurance companies to pay for *everything* but we ourselves don't want to pay for *anything*. Now that is a mathematical equation that will never add up.


### MALPRACTICE

I won't mince words. In my opinion, our current malpractice system is both immoral and intolerably inefficient. I call it immoral because it basically rewards those who have good lawyers and sympathetic juries with often outrageous awards while leaving the vast majority of people who are injured by complicated modern medical care out in the cold. (One journalist describes malpractice as a great legal lottery.) The current system is also terribly inefficient: Resolving liability and assessing compensation through the courts is expensive, time-consuming, and often does not deliver justice for the patient or the doctor involved.

According to one source, only about 2 percent of patients injured by substandard medical care actually file a malpractice claim—and only about a third of them actually receive any compensation through a settlement or trial. (Kendall, D. "Toolbox: Medical Malpractice Law Reform." *The American Interest*. Vol. 3, Number 3; Jan-Feb 2008. http://www.the-american-interest.com/article-bd.cfm?piece=387)

In fact, the actual cost of malpractice insurance premiums and awards is a relatively small part of overall health care expenditures—according to one estimate, about 2 percent. But the specter of being sued makes many doctors practice defensive medicine, and these indirect costs are much larger, leading to unnecessary expenses because "it's better to be safe than sorry." Estimates for these indirect costs range from fifty to hundreds of billions annually and no one can give a precise answer. But the number is significant, not only in actual dollar cost but in the emotional cost to doctors who are sometimes falsely accused in the hopes of a quick out-of-court settlement. No wonder a recent survey in the *Archives of Internal Medicine* indicates that 91 percent of American physicians practice defensive medicine by ordering tests that are not medically necessary (June 28, 2010).

In my opinion, the only sensible answer to this royal mess is some form of no-fault system—where *all* victims of injury, whether actual malpractice or not, are compensated according to living costs and projected lifespan through an impartial process using unbiased experts. Quite frankly I cannot understand the Democratic Party's reluctance to promote such reform, except as a matter of political pandering to the lawyer lobby. We must also have a foolproof process of identifying quickly and accurately those physicians who are truly incompetent—and promptly removing them from practice.

## MEDIA

Finally, I come to a powerful influence that obviously hits close to home. As I think about my own role in raising the public's health care expectations, I am vividly reminded of the reporting I did during the 1990s on the use of bone mar-row transplants for advanced breast cancer. Based on their own experience, many experts were advocating this costly and dangerous treatment. And, predictably, many insurance companies were denying payment saying that it was "experi-mental." The media were full of reports about greedy insur-ance companies and heartrending stories about women who were denied treatment (I did such a report during this pe-riod for ABC's *20/20*). But in 1999, at the annual meeting of international cancer experts, three double-blind, placebo-controlled trials (the gold-standard research trial) were pre-sented showing no difference in outcomes between the bone marrow treatment and standard chemotherapy. Almost over-night, doctors stopped doing these treatments. But in the meantime—because we had all (media, politicians, and ex-perts) jumped on the bandwagon without the proof of final studies—many women and their families had gone through unnecessary, costly, and dangerous treatment. (In this case, the insurance companies were right for the wrong reasons. The treatment was indeed "experimental," but often they were try-ing to save money for their bottom lines.)

## WASTE NOT, WANT NOT?

All these influences on spending quickly add up. Doctors, hospitals, pharmaceutical makers, insurance companies, the media, and consumers together create a lot of duplicative, wasteful care. In fact, many health care experts estimate that about *a third* of what we spend on health care is unnecessary. "Unnecessary" can include everything from outright fraud to treatment offered in good faith but for which there is no solid proof of benefit (like the bone marrow treatment just described). But let's do the math: *One-third of $2.6 trillion dollars comes to more than $800 billion wasted every year!* Given that it would cost about $300 billion to fully insure all of those in our country now uninsured, if we could actually prevent that unnecessary spending, we would have enough to insure everyone with money left over!

So why don't we go after that money? There are many reasons, but in my opinion, one of the most important is that the fruits of unnecessary spending are going to real people with real jobs. The money spent on unneeded treatments, aggressive sales and marketing, excessive paperwork, bonuses for insurance company executives, etc., may be deemed unnecessary to health care experts. But to the people working for that money, it pays the bills. It also puts money back into the general economy. Is it any wonder the health sector is the only major growing part of our economy? It now accounts for more than one-sixth of our entire GDP!

Understandably, politicians balk at getting rid of unnecessary health costs because they know it will also mean getting rid of real jobs. *That's why I have long believed that in order for us to realistically tackle the issue of medical waste we also have to address honestly the issue of the resultant job displacements.* We have to realize that some people will lose jobs if we truly reform our system, and we have to prepare for that by retraining such people for other jobs in health care—such as nurse practitioner, physician assistant, geriatric worker, and home health care worker—that will be needed to provide health care for our growing and older population.

So with all these forces driving up the costs of health care, is there any chance of bringing them under control? I have reluctantly come to the conclusion that there is only one possible answer—and I can predict that most of you are not going to like it initially. But, please, hear me out before you jump to any conclusion.

# CHAPTER THREE

# The Big Fear

I might as well lay it out right up front: In my opinion, there is no way to get costs and quality under control without a strong role for the federal government. Now, before you question my sanity, let me ask you this: Can you think of a private industry that is intensely competitive in the open marketplace but under the strong regulation of the federal government to the great benefit of all consumers? Answer: The airline industry.

You may be skeptical. Isn't the airline industry in a lot of trouble? Well, yes and no. Ironically, since the government deregulated the airline industry in 1978, the resulting intense competition has produced mixed results: lower prices but service that is less than ideal.

But there is one area where the government did *not* deregulate: the tight federal safety guidelines, which we all take for granted and would fight to the death to preserve. I think "fight to the death" is exactly the right phrase when talking about airplanes. Isn't it precisely our fear of dying in a crash that motivates us to support strong federal regulations that require pilots to be regularly re-certified and planes to be constantly inspected?

And in the case of the airlines, aren't you glad it is the federal government doing it, rather than fifty state governments independently setting their own safety standards for

planes and airports and pilots operating in their states? Isn't
it reassuring to know that the standards are uniform, no matter which airline or pilot, whether you are flying out of a small
airport in Wyoming or O'Hare in Chicago?

Contrast this airline regulation with the health care industry, where the hodgepodge of regulations and quality
controls can vary considerably from one hospital to another,
from one doctor to another, and from one state to another. The
lack of standardization is one reason why the independent
and prestigious Institute of Medicine (IOM) estimates that
there are as many as one hundred thousand deaths due to
medical errors in this country—every year! Can you imagine
if there were one hundred thousand deaths from airplane
crashes every year? Of course you can't, because we know
that the government would never let that happen; they would
shut down the industry immediately, after just a few crashes.

I start with this example in the high hopes that I can pique
your interest enough to read the rest of this chapter, where
I want to make a case for the essential role of the federal
government in health care. Notice I am not suggesting
any government "takeover," like the British system, where the
government literally owns and operates the hospitals and doctors. That would be a disaster in this country, in my opinion.
Rather I suggest an "essential role." So the question obviously
becomes what should that role be?

I will give you a big hint by suggesting it should be the
same kind of role the government plays in the Federal Employees Health Benefits (FEHB) program, sometimes called
the "Congressional Plan" because members of Congress participate in it.

## HOW CONGRESS IS CARED FOR

Actually, members of Congress have the same health insurance choices as other federal employees. Since Congress created the FEHB program in 1959, members of Congress and their staffs have had the same insurance choices as everyone else who works for (or retires from) the federal government. Now, that's not to say members of Congress don't get better medical care or have more advantages than average federal workers. (See below.) But as far as insurance coverage, the senior senator from, say, Illinois, is offered the same health insurance choices as the lowliest IRS desk clerk working in Peoria.

What stands out about the FEHB—and what makes it so different from most other employer health insurance programs—is the balance it strikes between choice and oversight.

If you are one of the nearly 160 million Americans who get their health insurance through their employer, then you probably aren't accustomed to having much of a choice when it comes to your health insurance. Many small companies offer only one option, usually an HMO provided by the only large insurance provider in the area. If you work for a really big company, you might have two or three choices—say a less expensive HMO, a more moderately priced PPO (preferred provider option), and a more costly fee-for-service plan—typically all provided by the same insurance carrier. Even if you are lucky enough to be offered a few choices, trying to understand and compare the types of benefits being offered and the costs for things like copays and deductibles is usually daunting, if not outright confusing.

The federal model is different, primarily because the federal government is so big. There are more than 8 million employees, retirees, and their family members in the FEHB program. (For comparison's sake, Walmart, the world's largest private employer, has fewer than 2 million workers—many of whom aren't even insured because they are part-time employees.)

Federal workers are spread out across every state, territory, and in most foreign countries. Their jobs vary from managing computer systems to inspecting meat; from maintaining national parks to arresting criminals. Forcing such a diverse group of employees to use the exact same private insurance plan would be logistically impossible.

To help deal with all of these people with different needs, the FEHB program is based on a simple idea called an insurance "exchange." Think of an exchange like a shopping mall. In this case, government manages the mall, decides each year what "stores" can sell their products in the mall, and sets some basic guidelines to make sure customers are treated fairly. But once allowed into the mall, the stores—in this example, the insurance companies—decide what they will sell and for how much. And the shoppers—in this case, federal workers—choose the products they want to buy based on quality and price.

The FEHB program is run by the Office of Personnel Management, or OPM. It's a fancy name, but it's basically the government's human resources department. OPM runs the massive FEHB program with a relatively small staff and for a comparatively low cost.

Each year OPM invites insurance companies in each state

to submit proposals. There are some ground rules. Insurers are not allowed to consider preexisting conditions or set waiting periods for health coverage to begin. They can't charge different prices depending on a participant's age, gender, or race; nor can they charge rates that are higher than the average cost of similar consumer plans being offered in the same state or region. Insurance companies must also offer basic services like prenatal and emergency room care. Other than these kinds of general rules, the benefits and services that the companies offer can vary widely—as can the prices they charge. Much like a private company does for its employees, the federal government pays a portion of each worker's or retiree's premium. Those who choose more expensive plans pay more out of their own pockets.

Here is where the ideas of private enterprise and competition come into the mix. Remember, in most private companies, workers rarely have any choice when it comes to their insurance plans. But because there are 8 million people in the FEHB program—which means 8 million monthly premiums to be paid—insurance companies really want to participate. The desire to participate is so strong that OPM is able to negotiate with the companies to keep their prices lower and their benefits stronger. Each year, about three hundred insurance companies participate in the program nationwide. That's a lot of choices for federal workers and retirees.

I should note that those choices do differ based on where federal employees live, mainly because insurance companies operate on a state-by-state basis. In places where there are lots of federal jobs, such as metropolitan Washington, DC, federal employees choose from as many as twelve different plans. In some smaller states, the choices are more limited. But over the years, the FEHB program has found a way to solve even that problem, by encouraging insurers to create a few nationwide plans. These national plans help make sure federal employees in even the most rural areas still have choices. Interestingly enough, what OPM has found is that because these national plans can spread their costs (or risk) out among so many federal workers, and because they don't have to worry about individual state rules, they typically provide the best value. In fact, almost half of all participants in the FEHB program are enrolled in the same national Blue Cross Blue Shield PPO plan!

By now I hope you're beginning to see why I like the FEHB program model. It gives people lots of choices but with very helpful and sensible government oversight.

And there's something else that makes the plan work really well: accessible information. Having a choice about your health insurance may sound great, but if you don't understand what you're choosing, you might make a bad decision. One thing the FEHB program does very well is to help participants understand what they are buying. OPM has pretty specific rules about how the various insurance plans must explain their benefits and costs. The plans in the program are required to use the same language and definitions. They all accept the same standard forms. There are online tools and a yearly book filled with detailed charts to help participants compare the costs and coverage. OPM also requires providers with more than five hundred subscribers to randomly survey the people they insure about their experience and satisfaction with a given plan. So, as part of their decision-making process, program participants can use this feedback as they compare insurance companies to each other. In sharing survey results such as "getting care quickly" and "how well doctors communicate," you can probably guess that plans with high costs and bad satisfaction ratings don't last very long!

The FEHB program is generally embraced by both ends of the political spectrum. Conservatives like that it is based on competition among private companies. Liberals like that the program is regulated by the government and prevents discrimination for things like age and preexisting conditions. And for many years, members of Congress have liked it because they get to say that they get the same care as every other federal employee!

Actually, that last point isn't quite accurate. It is true that members of Congress have the same *insurance* choices as all other federal workers, at least for now. That may change in 2014 under the new health care bill, when members of Congress might have to choose from the new state exchanges to be set up by then. But Congress does have a special bonus most people don't know about.

## THE HILL'S HEALTH BENEFIT BONUS

I think it's important to mention that members of Congress have access to an extra bonus when it comes to their own care. As part of my reporting for ABC News, I took a close look at this bonus. In fact, while members of Congress love to talk about the FEHB program, they do not like to discuss the medical clinic they use in the basement of the U.S. Capitol. It's called the Office of the Attending Physician (OAP), and it's staffed by some of the best doctors and nurses in the navy. Congress and the military fund it each year to the tune of several million dollars. The OAP provides emergency medical care to staff, visitors, and Congress members on Capitol Hill; coordinates vaccinations for overseas trips; and does physicals for the Capitol Police. But the office also provides members of Congress with a wealth of high-end medical care that no one else can get—all for a flat annual fee, currently around $500. For that low price, the Office brings in specialists for appointments with senators and House members; nurses do medical tests and X-rays; doctors write prescriptions and administer drugs. There are even therapists to coordinate physical therapy! On top of that, Congress has access to the VIP wings at military medical facilities in the Washington, DC, area, where they are given top-notch service.

I tried several times to schedule interviews with the Office of the Attending Physician to talk about these services, but my requests were turned down. (I even tried knocking on the door, and was asked to leave!) The Office refused to answer most of our questions on the basis of national security. Now, I don't begrudge members of Congress having access to this very convenient quality medical care. But I fear that having such care so readily available could prevent our leaders from truly understanding the issues that most

Americans face in trying to easily find quality care. I'd like to see everyone have access to similar care—to truly have "what Congress has"!

## LOOKING AHEAD TO THE 2014 EXCHANGE SYSTEM

The reason it is so important to understand what an exchange is—and is not—is that such exchanges, to be established at the state level by 2014, are at the heart of the new health bill. By now, you should understand that an exchange is a "place"— for most of us, it will be an Internet site—that allows you to choose an insurance plan that is best for you and/or your family. Like the federal employees' exchanges, the ones that are supposed to be available to many Americans by 2014 will compare insurance plans in plain English with no hidden conditions or costs. And because the insurance companies will be competing for your business, they should be offering the best possible deal they can and still survive financially. Obviously, it makes a big difference who is running these exchanges. At this point, you will not be surprised to read that I believe the federal government should set the basic rules and conditions. Whether or not the states will be able to run the exchanges on a day-to-day basis depends on how the whole system is structured, but in my view, the Federal Government has to play a strong role in order to guarantee that all insurance companies play by the same rules and standards. It is ultimately the only way that all of our citizens can be offered a level playing field when they try to buy insurance.

At this point, I think it would be informative to look at another large industrialized country that has implemented this idea of the federal government as a regulator of private insurance, in a somewhat different way. I have chosen Germany because it is the largest economy in Europe and intensely capitalistic in orientation.

### WHAT WE MIGHT LEARN FROM GERMANY

Germany has accomplished universal health coverage (99.8 percent of its citizens have health insurance) through private, nonprofit insurance companies under government regulation. All Germans have guaranteed access to medical care and premiums are based on ability to pay. And those who can't afford to pay at all have their benefits paid for by various government programs. Regardless, everyone gets the same health coverage—everyone. This concept, termed "social solidarity," remains the guiding principle in Germany's health care system.

The key players in this system are *nonprofit, nongovernment* insurance plans, called "sickness or statutory funds." Approximately 90 percent of Germans participate in this system (the remaining 10 percent obtain coverage through private insurance plans). Currently, there are about 170 sickness funds to choose from—and the key is that Germans choose based on whichever fund best suits their individual needs or is perceived to have the best services. They do not choose based on cost, because the funds all cost the same for the same services and provide the same minimum benefits package.

The system works because all Germans are required by law to have health insurance for hospital and outpatient medical care. For individuals earning less than $64,000 per year, participation in one of the government regulated plans is mandatory. Those earning more than $64,000 are free to enroll in the sickness fund of their choice or separately purchase health care insurance from one of the fifty private insurance plans available (private insurance companies must also provide minimum benefit packages). Those who want just a little more than the sickness funds offer can purchase a supplemental plan from one of the private companies. Neither the sickness funds nor the private insurance plans can deny coverage to anyone with a preexisting condition or drop patients if they become ill.

Health care costs are paid by premiums based on 15.5 percent of a worker's gross pay; employees pay 8.2 percent and employers pay 7.3 percent (even for those Germans who opt to purchase private insurance). Premiums are deposited in a central national fund. Prior to 2009, the standard employee/employer contribution also covered dependent children. Now all children are covered by tax dollars from the federal government, without additional charge to employees or employers. In an effort to be more prepared for the expense of caring for Germany's aging population, all Germans are also required to purchase long-term nursing care insurance (2.2 percent of a worker's gross pay, with half paid by the employee and half by the employer).

The central fund, now stocked with premiums paid by

employees and employers, then pays a set rate directly to the sickness fund to cover the entirety of an individual's medical costs. The dollar amount paid to the sickness fund for a given person is risk-adjusted for age, gender, and eighty chronic conditions. Each fund then has to make do with the allocated amount to pay and care for that individual. Funds form associations with each other for negotiating purposes and then negotiate with physician groups and drug companies to determine reimbursement rates. The federal government provides a framework for the negotiations and ensures all parties stick to set prices for disease management and prevention.

Sickness funds do well—and therefore attract more patients and more money from the central government fund—when they please their members with quality, cost-effective care. If a sickness fund finds itself with money woes, the fund must either adjust its spending or charge its subscribers additional premiums (up to a maximum of 2 percent of wages) to break even. Funds that find themselves in a deficit are then forced to allow their subscribers the option of leaving the fund at the end of the year.

Conversely, sickness funds that are in the fortunate (but rare) situation of having money left over after paying for the health care of all their members don't line their pockets with these profits; sickness funds are "nonprofit." The extra money is either used to provide additional benefits or can be returned to members as a rebate. The funds are pitted against one another—efficient funds that provide high-quality care and stay under budget are rewarded with more enrollees in years to come, while poor-performing funds will gradually be pushed out of the market.

Although the sickness fund coverage option is popular, 10 percent of Germans opt out, because they are either wealthy or self-employed. These people (who are still required to have health insurance) purchase private, for-profit, commercial health insurance, similar to the plans available here. Patients enjoy certain luxuries, including a wider choice of medical and dental treatments, private hospital rooms, and quicker access to top-notch doctors, and doctors earn higher reimbursements from privately insured patients.

Government regulation to maintain quality, cost-effective universal insurance is enforced through a joint federal committee (JFC) which is the supreme and legally binding decision-making body for the country's health care enterprise. The JFC has wide-ranging regulatory powers and is tasked with making evidence-based coverage decisions regarding innovations and determining benefit packages and reimbursements. The JFC is composed of representatives of all parts of the health care industry, including patients. Absolutely key is that regulation, negotiation oversight, and medical policy decision making is done by JFC experts—including hospitals, doctors, patients, the sickness funds themselves, and mutually agreed on neutral parties—*not* by politicians subject to lobbying pressure!

In conjunction with the JFC, the government has also created an Institute for Quality and Cost Effectiveness to evaluate the quality and effectiveness of medical care and drugs. This organization objectively determines the advantages and disadvantages of medical services available to German patients and then makes independent recommendations to the JFC based on studies comparing various drugs, tests, treatments, etc. The Institute for Quality and Cost Effectiveness publishes all of its reports on a user-friendly resource website available to providers and patients. Effective chronic disease management, which incorporates coordination of care, is rewarded via financial incentives to sickness funds, higher reimbursements for physicians, and lower copays for patients.

Virtually every German has insurance coverage at a much lower per person cost than in the United States. (The latest figures: $3,737 per person in Germany in 2008 vs. $8086 in 2009 in the U.S.) Germans say that happens because they avoid expensive emergency room care traditionally used by the uninsured and because patients with insurance seek care earlier and do not forgo care because of cost restraints. Also, the collective bargaining power of large pools of patients in the sickness funds helps keep costs down. Finally, because the entire health care process is more streamlined in Germany, administrative costs are also much lower than in America (6 percent in Germany compared to 13.7 percent for private insurance companies in the United States).

One looming problem: Doctors are not as well paid in Germany as in the United States and collectively feel undervalued. They went to the picket lines in 2006, albeit in vain. Having said that, it's important to know also that medical school tuition is essentially free in Germany.

No health system is perfect, and despite government oversight and universal coverage, in the summer of 2010 Germans were faced with health insurance rate hikes (from 14.9 percent to 15.5 percent of gross pay) to combat a $13.8 billion deficit in the public health insurance system. Germany also recognizes areas in need of improvement, including increased funding for medical research, translation of medical advances to the bedside, and better chronic disease management and prevention.

After reading about Germany, you should have a better sense of how a federal government can serve as the national regulator of the private health insurance industry.

## HOW OUR GOVERNMENT IS ALREADY
## INVOLVED IN HEALTH CARE

Our federal government already plays important roles in our health care. For example, in Medicare, the federal government is both the actual insurer (for people over sixty-five) as well as a regulator. In Medicare, the government, as the only insurer, actually collects the money (through taxes and the relatively low premiums paid by senior citizens) and pays the bills submitted by doctors and hospitals directly to Medicare. Medicare patients can still choose whatever doctors and hospitals they want. While Medicare is the insurer, it is not the owner and operator of the doctors and hospitals. Think of it this way: Medicare is like the Canadian health care system, where the government (via the individual provinces) serves as the insurer but patients can choose their own private doctors and hospitals. And both Medicare and the Canadian system are very different from Great Britain, where the government functions as the insurer (paying the bills) *and* also owns the doctors and hospitals. Now that is true socialized medicine!

## OUR SECRET "SOCIALIZED" MEDICINE

Believe it or not, we have an example of true socialized medicine in this country! It's the VA (Veterans Administration) health care system. If I wanted to write a provocative headline, it could legitimately be this one: CONGRESS SUPPORTS SOCIALIZED MEDICINE FOR OUR VETERANS. That headline would be true because:

1. The VA system is owned and operated by the federal government through the Department of Veterans Affairs. The doctors and hospitals in the VA system work for the government. And the government decides how the doctors and hospitals should be practicing and providing medicine for our veterans.
2. Congress (some members reluctantly) supports this system because they know the vast majority of vets who use it are very pleased with it. The VA system is now regarded by many as the best health care system in the country in terms of providing quality care at a reasonable cost.

Another government option to understand is the so-called "public option," advocated by President Obama (and many others) during his campaign. Put very simply, it would be similar to a Medicare-type insurance program for people *under* sixty-five. It would be a government-run insurance program and would allow patients to choose their own doctors and hospitals. It would *not* be government-run like the

VA system (see previous box, "Our Secret 'Socialized' Medicine").

So why are so many so emotionally opposed to a public option? Private insurance companies are vigorously opposed because they know it would be difficult, if not impossible, to compete against such an option. Private insurance companies have to pay for overhead costs that the government does not, such as salaries for salespersons, marketing and advertising expenses, returns to stockholders, much larger bonuses. According to one analysis, the overhead costs for private, for-profit insurers average about 11.7 percent, compared to 1.3 percent for Medicare.

Obviously the private insurers and their political allies have succeeded in convincing most Americans that a public option would be a government takeover or, even worse, socialized medicine. But the public option would basically be a Medicare-like choice, in which the government pays the bills but choice of providers is left up to the consumer. Thus, it is neither a government takeover nor socialized medicine. In fact, anyone who insists on using these labels for a "public option" would also have to label Medicare as socialized medicine!

So does this mean I favor a public option? If I had a magic wand and could redesign our health care from scratch, I would recommend "Medicare for All"—in other words, a public option as the only insurance choice for everyone. My reasons for saying this are strictly pragmatic, not political. I believe the potential efficiency of a single-payer system (like Medicare) would ultimately save many billions (the differential in overhead between Medicare and the private insurance industry). That money could be used to pay for actual health care rather than overhead. And this system would preserve private health care delivery (freedom of choice for consumers), but in a much more regulated and truly competitive fashion. Private insurers could no longer confuse us with their cost and coverage options. "Medicare for All" would also have the clout to deal directly with the other drivers of health care costs, such as drug companies, malpractice lawyers, and the media.

But politically, I don't think this is possible. The idea has been effectively demonized by its opponents—that is, the politicians acting on behalf of private, for-profit insurance companies and their lobbyists. And, to be honest, I believe that the private insurance companies' fears—that competing directly against the nonprofit public option would price them out of the market—are legitimate. I don't see how they could compete, with their much higher overhead, including the necessity to make profits for their stockholders.

Tough luck, you may think. If they can't compete, they shouldn't be in business. Isn't that what free marketplace forces are all about? But putting the private insurers completely out of business would mean a tremendous dislocation of people and jobs in our already fragile economy. One politically possible compromise might be a system similar to Germany's, where the federal government sets up the framework in which private insurance companies compete in an honest and understandable marketplace. (Remember: Germany does not have a public option as part of its insurance mix; that's proof that health care costs and quality can be somewhat controlled without a public option *if* the government regulates the private insurance market in a sensible way.) In terms of political philosophy, I'd describe this as a "side-by-side" arrangement of government and private insurance rather than "top-down," as is the case in Great Britain. And if a large, capitalistic country like Germany can do it, why can't we?

If done right, this kind of partnership between government and the private sector would mean that we, the consumers, become empowered to make real choices. It would mean that insurers would have to compete for our business on the basis of service, not hidden financial tricks, because they would all have to play by the same rules. That means that once a year— like Germany—we could fire our insurance company if they didn't treat us right. Now, I ask you, what's wrong with that?

But what are the chances of that actually happening in this country? Are we morally responsible for one another, in sickness and in health? Next chapter, please.

# CHAPTER FOUR

# The Big Sermon

Up to this point, we've focused on the economic and political aspects of health care, but I also think it is important to explore the moral issues related to it. The most basic question, of course, is whether or not we have a moral obligation to provide health care for all our citizens.

Actually, polls show that most Americans feel we should not let people die on the streets, and that we should take care of them when they "really need it." The debates start when we try to discuss how to fulfill this obligation. Should we do it like we do now, with multiple levels of care, where those with money and/or good insurance can get attention more readily and earlier than those who don't have those resources? What's wrong with that as long as everyone eventually gets care? (As then-president George W. Bush once said, we have "access to care" because anyone can "just go to the emergency room.")

Well, there are several problems with this approach. One is economic. People without health insurance tend to delay getting care. When they finally get into the system, usually through the emergency room, their care will often be more complicated and costly than if they could have been treated at an earlier stage—or if their illness could have been prevented in the first place. The uninsured account for about one-fifth of ER visits in this country.

Take the example of an early stage pneumonia: Those of us with good insurance and ready access to some kind of primary care will get it treated with antibiotics—if it is caused by bacteria—but a person without insurance may delay to the point where they need to be admitted to the ICU with pulmonary failure, at which point their pneumonia may cost hundreds of thousands of dollars to treat.

So here's the point: If we are going to treat everyone eventually, when they get sick enough, why not provide basic insurance that would encourage people to get care earlier? We do have universal *care* in the sense that we usually don't let people die on the street. What we need is universal *insurance coverage* that provides preventive care and treatment at an earlier stage. I agree with those experts who point out that *it is no accident that every other developed country has universal coverage* and *at significantly lower cost per person than the United States.*

And we should never forget that those of us fortunate enough to have health insurance are, in fact, already helping to pay for those who don't have it—we just don't see it directly on our bills. Somebody has to pay, one way or another, for all the care provided in emergency rooms and public clinics for the uninsured. Most of that cost is paid by federal, state, and local governments—and ultimately by U.S. taxpayers. Another way the uninsured are paid for is "cost shifting," in which hospitals charge higher prices to those with private insurance to help pay for the uninsured. So, again, if we are going to take care of the uninsured anyway (and pay for it), why not do it up front through direct insurance coverage, where the money spent could be more effective?

That's why I also favor mandates requiring everyone to buy health insurance—presuming it is priced fairly and that subsidies are available for those who truly cannot afford it. Again, if we can get over the emotional reaction of not liking "the government telling us what to do," insurance mandates make sense at several levels.

First, the basic idea of all insurance is to spread the risk as widely as possible. The more people paying into the insurance pool, the lower the cost for everyone. Second, it is also the fair thing to do. People who are young and healthy often complain about paying for something they don't need. But when they do get sick or have an accident and end up in the ER, they usually expect to be taken care of by "society."

What about the "moral hazard" argument, which basically says that if you give people something for free or very cheaply, they will abuse the offer? A bowl of candy that is free, for example, will disappear more quickly than one where you have to pay by the piece. And some experts predict that is what will happen with universal health insurance coverage: People will abuse it by going to the doctor or clinic at the slightest twinge of pain. Clearly, this is a potential problem, which is why almost everyone agrees there has to be some sensible system of copays to prevent frivolous decisions. But aside from true hypochondriacs, my guess is that not many people will abuse the system for unnecessary major treatments or tests.

## INSURANCE FOR ALL:
## A LIFE-OR-DEATH ISSUE

For me, the lack of good health insurance becomes a moral issue because we now have good data to show that people without insurance have a higher risk of premature death than those with it. *A recent Harvard study suggests that as many as forty-five thousand people in this country die prematurely every year because they lack health insurance.* How can people who call themselves "pro-life" live with that? I find it absolutely unacceptable as well as embarrassing that a country as rich as ours is the only developed country in the world without universal coverage!

But if economics and deaths don't move you, what about religious teachings? As an ordained Protestant minister (I finished seminary before starting medical school), I am going to briefly describe two parables told by Jesus of Nazareth as recorded in the New Testament. (There are many more passages I could refer to, but these two make my point.)

**1. The Parable of the Good Samaritan:** Parables are stories told to make a moral point. This one was told by Jesus in response to a question from someone described as a "teacher of the Law" who had asked what he must do "to inherit eternal life." In response, Jesus quoted the great commandment from Hebrew Scripture, "Love the Lord your God with all your heart and with all your soul and with all your strength and with all your mind—and love your neighbor as yourself." At which point, the teacher of the Law asked Jesus, "Who is my neighbor?" Jesus tells the following parable—one that has a particular bite to it, because Samaritans were often disliked for their lack of religious orthodoxy:

> There once was a man who was going down from Jerusalem to Jericho when robbers attacked him, stripped him, and beat him up, leaving him half-dead. It so happened that a priest was going down that road; but when he saw the man, he walked on by on the other side. In the same way a Levite also came there, went over, and looked at the man, and then walked on by on the other side. But a Samaritan who was traveling that way came upon the man, and when he saw him his heart was filled with pity. He went over to him, poured oil and wine on his wounds and then bandaged them; then he took him to an inn, where he took care of him. The next day he took out two silver coins and gave them to the innkeeper. "Take care of him," he told the innkeeper, "and when I come back this way, I will pay you whatever else you spend on him."

> And Jesus concluded, "In your opinion, which one of these three acted like a neighbor toward the man attacked by the robbers?"
> The teacher of the Law answered, "The one who was kind to him."
> Jesus replied, "You go, then, and do the same."

I could find no better way of expressing what this parable says to me than the words of two Boston physicians in their

1810 petition to start a new hospital for that city's most needy. To justify their petition they said:

> When in distress every man becomes our neighbor, not only if he be of the household of faith, but even though his misfortunes have been induced by transgressing the rules both of reason and religion.

That petition led to the formation of Boston's first public hospital in 1821. Now, almost 200 years later, that hospital is the world famous Massachusetts General Hospital, and it continues its mission of treating all those brought to its doors as "neighbors" regardless of their financial or social circumstances.

**2. The Parable of Final Judgment:** Most scholars believe that this was the final parable told by Jesus; it certainly has the feel of "last times." Here it is:

> When the Son of Man comes as King and all the angels with him, he will sit on his royal throne, and the people of all the nations will be gathered before him. Then he will divide them into two groups, just as a shepherd separates the sheep from the goats. He will put the righteous people at his right and the others at his left.
>
> Then the King will say to the people on his right, "Come, you that are blessed by my Father! Come and possess the kingdom which has been prepared for you ever since the creation of the world. I was hungry and

you fed me, thirsty and you gave me a drink; I was a stranger and you received me in your homes, naked and you clothed me; I was sick and you took care of me, in prison and you visited me."

The righteous will then answer him, "When, Lord, did we ever see you hungry and feed you, or thirsty and give you a drink? When did we ever see you a stranger and welcome you in our homes, or naked and clothe you? When did we ever see you sick and take care of you, or in prison, and visit you?"

The King will reply, "I tell you, whenever you did this for one of the least important of these brothers of mine, you did it for me!"

To me, this parable means that when we do basic acts of kindness for no ulterior reward or motive, we are also doing God's work. And for those of us who claim to be Christians, or as I prefer to call myself, a follower of Jesus, I think the meaning of these passages is inescapable when it comes to health care. *I believe it is impossible to be both a true follower of Jesus (or many other religious leaders and prophets) without also advocating basic health care for all.* Now I again recognize that there is a legitimate debate about *how* to accomplish this, but there should be no debate about *whether* to do it.

Of course, I recognize that many Americans are not religious or may not feel any such motivation. But there is much in our national history and psyche to suggest that we are a country that is indeed founded on a commitment to "life, liberty and the pursuit of happiness," as stated in the Declaration of Independence. So I ask very simply: How can anyone be assured of the pursuit of happiness, let alone life and liberty, without reasonable access to good health care?

What is the moral difference between guaranteeing basic police and fire protection versus guaranteeing basic health protection? We would never parcel out police and fire safety according to income levels or deny it because of preexisting conditions. But we do that all the time with health care.

What about the ultimate economic argument that we simply can't afford to provide basic health insurance for all our citizens, and that given our current deficits, this added cost would be a budget breaker? By now, you should know that I believe such an argument cannot be politically or economically correct *given that every other developed country in the world provides universal health insurance coverage at a lower per-person cost!!!* I believe that it is the right thing to do, both morally and economically. So the real question becomes, why aren't we doing it? Time for the Big Prediction.

# CHAPTER FIVE

# The Big Prediction

Without further ado—*here it is:*

NO DEVELOPED COUNTRY—INCLUDING THE UNITED STATES—WILL BE ABLE TO PAY FOR EVERY-THING FOR EVERYONE AT EVERY AGE THAT MODERN MEDICAL SCIENCE MIGHT DREAM UP.

Every developed country will be struggling with health care costs as their populations live longer and consequently develop more illnesses. The United States is right now in big-ger trouble than other countries because we already spend so much more. So we Americans need to have an honest discus-sion about our very real problems and possible solutions—free of political and partisan slogans that cover our problems with platitudes or falsehoods. This chapter is my attempt to contribute to this desperately needed dialogue.

Because it is ultimately financially impossible to provide all the latest and costly care to everyone at every age, all de-veloped countries will have to make some hard choices about what they *can* afford to provide to their citizens. Another word for "hard choices," of course, is "rationing." It's no longer a question of whether we have to engage in rationing, but only a question of how and when. Will the rationing be *ratio-nal* (as described earlier in Germany, based on objective deci-sions derived from effectiveness data) or *irrational* (as now so often occurs in this country, based on an individual's wealth and/or insurance combined with the person's ability to navigate the system and find good care).

Based on our *current* health care practices, here is my prediction for the United States in particular: *No matter what legislation Congress develops this year or in the years to come, health care costs will continue to rise. Within five to ten years, health care costs will be so out of control that we—the public—will demand that the government bail us out. At that point, the easiest and quickest action will be to expand Medicare to cover everyone.* The reason that will be so appealing in the face of economic disaster is that the control of costs would be in one place—the government. You may not like this prediction, but I am willing to bet my life savings that it will happen—*unless* we act decisively to change the way we now do business in health care.

There is one scientific possibility that *might* impact this dire prediction: If modern medical science can find simple and pervasive cures at the cellular level (using the exploding knowledge we are gaining from genetics and molecular biology), that *could* have an enormous impact on the costs of preventing, screening, and treating major illnesses, such as various types of cancer and heart disease. For example, if we could figure out what makes cells grow out of control (the common denominator in all cancers), we might then have a simple answer for all cancers, not our current variety of individual treatments for each cancer. Or if we could find the basis for atherosclerosis—the process underlying fatty buildup in our arteries—then we might avoid the costly angioplasties and bypass surgeries now required. I am not holding my breath, but these kinds of discoveries are certainly theoretically possible.

But short of such miraculous developments, there are some critical problems we can and should address. I don't pretend to have easy or even not-so-easy answers. But as is the case in patient care, I do know that we will never find the right answers unless we make the right diagnoses. And the right diagnoses are not possible unless we are willing to honestly address the symptoms and face the truth. Here is my list of the most important problems we need to address, along with some attempts at answers.

## PAYMENT REFORM

Our current "system" is a chaotic collection of public and private insurance plans that deal with a bewildering array of providers ranging from outstanding urban medical centers to individual practitioners and small hospitals in remote rural areas—and everything imaginable in between. If Medicare became the sole *insurer* in this country, we would finally have a truly national *insurance system* that would have the clout to change many of the problems I have discussed in this book. But in order for even that drastic step to work, we would have to make major reforms to Medicare, reforms that need to be made right now, given that Medicare accounts for about 20 percent of our total annual health care expenditure.

*The most basic reform needed is a change in the way we pay providers.* We need to remove the incentive to simply do more to make more—which is what the current fee-for-service payment system encourages.

A very dramatic example of this perverse payment system

is described in the June 20, 2010, issue of the *New York Times Magazine*. A writer named Katy Butler relates a literally heart-breaking saga (titled "My Father's Broken Heart") in which her father is urged to get a sophisticated heart pacemaker. Her aged mother is told that her husband needs the pacemaker for a slow heart rate that might kill him. She is told this despite the fact that his life had already been devastated by a major stroke at age seventy-nine. But the doctor, the hospital, and the device maker all had a financial stake in pushing the pacemaker—collectively, they would be paid more than $13,000 by Medicare for doing the procedure. Butler's father had the procedure done and lived another five years in a bed-ridden, senile state. When he finally died of pneumonia, the pacemaker was still working, and it had to be cut out before they could cremate his body, lest it explode from the heat of cremation!

Given these kinds of stories, which occur every day in this country, it's important to remember that an earlier ver-sion of the new health care reform bill would have provided payment for independent experts to discuss these kinds of decisions with patients and families *before* they were made. But that provision was labeled a "death panel" and removed.

Now, to be fair, the reform bill that did pass does have some provisions to move us toward payment reform. For ex-ample, a new Center for Medicare and Medicaid Innovation is supposed to encourage experiments in new ways of paying for outcomes rather than for services. (This provision sup-ports *local* experiments and is not a federal government take-over of health care, as is so often charged by critics.)

Another example is an Independent Payment Advisory

Board for controlling Medicare spending. (All experts agree that changes in Medicare are important not only because of their immediate effect on Medicare itself, but also because private insurers tend to follow Medicare's lead when it comes to key changes.) According to the current bill (which can always be changed by future legislation), the president would nominate the fifteen members of the board and the Senate would have to confirm. The board could put its proposals into effect *unless Congress objected within thirty days.* (The president could veto any objections and it would take a two-thirds majority of both houses of Congress to override the veto.)

However, the ultimate authority for Medicare would still reside with Congress, and I think it will be very tempting for Congress to interfere on behalf of various special interests who are, in their own narrow view, being negatively affected by attempts at payment reform. In my opinion, for true reform to occur, Congress would have to cede critical decision-making and operating power to a group of independent experts that is free of day-to-day political and lobbying pressure—and not subject to easy interference by Congress. (Remember: During the recent reform debate, there were approximately eight health care lobbyists for each member of Congress!)

## INDEPENDENT EXPERTS

I believe the only chance of real payment reform before hitting the crisis point described above involves getting health care reform out of the hands of the politicians—whose partisan juices and fear of voters paralyzes them from doing any real reform. So if we take reform out of their hands, whose hands should we trust?

Like others, I support the idea of an independent board of experts, somewhat analogous to the Federal Reserve for the banking system or the FAA for the airline industry. This board would have representation from all parts of the health care enterprise, including consumers, and would have responsibilities for the hard decisions—such as national standards for information technology, outcomes research, resource allocation, and safety standards and regulation.

Once this National Health Board is operative, it could establish and coordinate the crucial elements of any true reform—including these four:

**1. National IT (Information Technology) Standards:** It is impossible to establish all the other needed parts of true *national* reform without a national IT standard that any and all parts of American health care can use. Every currently successful health care system in this country is built around a functioning computer system that makes it easy to share data, records, etc.

Unfortunately, according to a 2009 *New England Journal of Medicine* study, only 1.5 percent of hospitals and 4 percent of doctors met the standard of a fully comprehensive record system. The federal government has designated $19 billion toward helping doctors and hospitals, so I am hopeful there will finally be significant movement on this front.

**2. Comparative Outcomes Research:** As we have seen in our brief look at health care in Germany (Chapter 3), some kind of government program to support study of the comparative effectiveness of existing and new treatments, drugs, devices, etc., is essential in making rational decisions about what insurance should pay for. We have to have solid research on what value we get for our health care dollars in order to make rational spending decisions. There have been past attempts to do this in the United States, but they have been fought tooth and nail by the parts of the "medical industrial" complex affected. That's one reason an independent group of experts must be empowered to make these kinds of decisions.

The new legislation does create a nonprofit Patient-Centered Outcomes Research Institute, which is supposed to study the "relative health outcomes, clinical effectiveness, and appropriateness" of various medical maneuvers, both by evaluating old studies and doing their own. However—and I think this is very telling—the legislation specifically prohibits this institute from using their results to make actual decisions about coverage or reimbursement rates. So unless some other group/agency is given the authority to use this data to make these decisions, it may be nothing more than a paper tiger. Optimists think that once this data is available, it will be used by Medicare and private insurers to guide their decisions; pessimists—who seem to have history on their side—think this institute will eventually be emasculated by special interests.

**3. Emphasis on Primary Care:** But even with nationally available computer technology—and consequent access to data about what works and what doesn't—coordinated care to use these resources effectively will not be possible without adequate primary care.

As I pointed out earlier, in previous generations this kind

of care was provided by GPs who were trained to at least initially treat all members of a family, from newborns to the elderly. Obviously, as medical information and technology expanded exponentially, that kind of care became impossible for a single doctor to provide, hence the explosion of specialists. But as we all know, some vital things were lost in the transition from the family doctor to the laundry list of specialists—one of the most important of which was the *coordination* of our care, especially for complicated problems.

Currently, approximately 30 percent of our doctors are in primary care and 70 percent are specialists. And the number of new doctors choosing primary care (family physicians, general internists, and pediatricians) has been steadily dropping. That is in stark contrast to most other developed countries, where the split is closer to fifty-fifty.

There are many reasons why most medical problems can and should be handled by primary care doctors—and their invaluable colleagues known as physician assistants and nurse practitioners. At least according to current payment practices, primary care providers usually charge less, even for the same services. More importantly for patient satisfaction and safety, *primary care providers* (I will now use that phrase to include primary care physicians, nurse practitioners, and physician assistants) typically are the ones who keep track of a given person's medical history—and coordinate the input from various specialists, including all the drugs prescribed by various doctors. This absolutely vital function typically falls through the cracks when too many specialists are involved.

That's exactly what happened in the case of the pacemaker insertion I briefly described earlier. The stroke victim's elderly wife was pushed by a cardiologist to have the pacemaker inserted. Their family physician, who knew them well and might have talked them out of the procedure, was notified by fax—*after* the procedure had been done!

And here is another example that is even more dramatic because it demonstrates the terrible consequences that can result from the lack of basic coordination in modern health care. In his speech to the 2010 graduating class at Stanford Medical School, Atul Gawande, the brilliant physician-writer for *The New Yorker*, told the story of a thirty-four-year-old patient who suffered multiple, life-threatening injuries in an auto accident. Because he was fortunate to end up in the care of a skilled trauma team, his life was saved by spectacular specialists doing their magic. However, that same setting—an array of specialists focused on their own tasks—also cost him all his toes and fingers. No, doctors didn't miss seeing that his digits were in need of treatment; they were not injured in the accident. But no one gave him the vaccines required to prevent future infections because his ruptured spleen had been removed. Everyone taking care of him had to have known that he needed the vaccines. But no individual doctor/nurse/administrator had the specific responsibility to make sure this was done before he left the hospital. That's what a good primary doctor should do in a true system that coordinates the care provided by specialists. So two years later, while on vacation, this man whose life had been saved by modern medical care, picked up a strep infection that took over his body because of the missed vaccines, and he had to have his toes and fingers amputated. That devastating infection should never have happened with truly coordinated care.

So how do we make primary care more attractive to graduating medical students? Most other developed countries do it by a combination of various incentives that:

- make pay more equivalent to specialists
- provide subsidies and other support for students who choose primary care (including forgiveness of student loans or paying for medical school tuition in the first place)
- improve working conditions (hours, coverage, etc.) for primary care providers

**4. The Medical Home:** This phrase is increasingly used to describe an actual place/office/clinic where patients can go for their primary care; not just diagnosis and treatment, but a lifelong program of prevention, early screening, and chronic condition management. Ideally, it is staffed by primary care providers. The goal is to provide care quickly and efficiently and to avoid the more costly and inefficient emergency room as a substitute for true primary care.

The new reform legislation does include approximately $11 billion to support community health centers in low-income areas. Presumably, these community centers will function as medical homes; this money could turn out to be very well spent if it achieves the goal of cutting down on emergency room use.

In order to operate optimally, these medical homes need to function as part of an overall system that provides coordinated specialty care when needed. The world famous Mayo Clinic had to learn this the hard way when they discovered that too many of their employees were going to the emergency room because they couldn't get appointments with primary care doctors in the Mayo system. So the clinic spent the money to hire more primary care doctors and nurse practitioners. This coordinated combination of primary and specialty care has both improved care and saved money.

Obviously the above are only the bare bones of what is needed in truly comprehensive health care reform. But I mention these four as examples of vital change that I believe can only be accomplished by direction and decision-making at the national level.

And I would remind you of some of the many possible shorter-term improvements that I have discussed throughout the book, including:

**1. Creating Health Insurance Exchanges (Chapter 3):** By providing the setting for real competition between insurance companies, exchanges could help control costs and provide better choices. Unfortunately, under the current bill, these state exchanges are not scheduled to become operative until 2014; I would strongly urge government planners to push up that starting date as much as possible.

**2. Reforming Medical Malpractice (Chapter 2):** This is something that can and should be done almost immediately. All it requires is the moral and political will to do what everyone—except lawyers and their supporters, mostly Democrats—knows should be done.

**3. Better Study of New Drugs and Devices (Chapter2):** These changes in the way the FDA operates can be done quickly if the agency is given the proper authority and resources by Congress.

## WHAT'S IT GOING TO TAKE?

These kinds of changes, and the longer-term ones I have described in this chapter, require two ingredients that have been in short supply:

**1. Political Leadership:** Nothing significant in health care reform will happen without a president and Congress who are willing to put political *courage* above political *expediency*. Some would argue that President Obama has already done that—by pushing for needed reforms even though they are currently unpopular with many Americans.

**2. Personal Sacrifice:** As I said in Chapter 2, this is the toughest nut to crack—the unrealistic expectation that we Americans can have everything we want or think we need without bankrupting ourselves and the country. But the good news is that *more is not always better.*

If we can learn how to accept just what we truly need for good health care, it will not only usually cost less, but will often produce better results. In other words, the latest and most dramatic treatments are often not what *are* really best for us. We need both health care leaders and primary care facilities that can provide us with the information to make the right choices. I am convinced that if we had that kind of honest and understandable information, we would make the right choices most of the time.

So I end this primer on what we should know about the current and possible future status of American health care with a good news/bad news prediction.

The good news is that the newly passed health care bill should eventually provide some kind of health insurance (devilish details still to come) to more than 30 million Americans now uninsured. The bad news is that the bill does not provide any assured ways of controlling costs and guaranteeing quality. I do believe that some of the proposed boards and experiments to control costs will result in some sporadic and modest improvements, but I believe the political and economic pressures (for jobs and profits) from the medical-industrial complex will override truly significant cost control. Therefore, I predict the government will have to bail us out by expanding Medicare to cover everyone. As I have pointed out, there is nothing immediately magical about "Medicare for All"—Medicare itself needs major reform—but it does offer the possibility of true national reforms because it is a *national insurance* system.

I hope I am wrong. I would love to see the "public-private partnership" concept I have described earlier in countries like Germany take hold here—where the federal government, with guidance from all levels of health care, sets the rules and framework within which the private sector vigorously competes for our business.

But I have to wonder whether we Americans will be willing

to support the necessary changes in time to slow down health care cost increases in any significant way; we tend to focus primarily on our own wants/desires without considering their impact on the big picture. The best (or worst) example of that is the way we continue to overeat, drink, and smoke even while knowing how bad they are for our health.

Our current attitudes about petroleum products are another telling example: We know that our dependency on these products is unsustainable (the same word we use for growing health care costs), but we want somebody else to make the necessary sacrifices and changes. We seem to be a country that does not take decisive action on any major social problem (civil rights, home mortgages, immigration, education reform) until our backs are against the proverbial wall. So if you forced me to bet, right now I would have to bet against the possibility of true national health care reform in the short run, especially effective and fair cost control.

However, my generation will survive the coming catastrophe. I can only hope that our children will be wiser than we have been—and the reality is that they will have no choice other than a major government intervention *if we don't start true reform now.* The problems—and solutions—are, as usual, within ourselves.